THE VAGUS NERVE GUT WONDER HANDBOOK

THE A-Z TO ACTIVATE GUT HEALTH BY HEALING YOUR VAGUS NERVE

By

Dr. Chris Allan

TABLE OF CONTENTS

INTRODUCTION

Deep within your center sits the vagus nerve, a remarkable neurological highway that connects your brain to your gut and influences every element of your health and vitality. Often undervalued, this remarkable nerve plays a key part in your physical, mental, and emotional wellness.

In this breakthrough book, we go deep into the labyrinthine paths of the vagus nerve, uncovering its remarkable potential to:

◆ Relieve Stress and Anxiety: Discover simple strategies to activate your vagus nerve's relaxing influence, providing peace in the craziness of modern life.

- Boost Digestive Health: Uncover the vagus nerve's role as your body's natural digestive maestro, promoting optimal gut health, and digestion.

- Enhance Immunity: Learn how to bolster your immune system's defenses by leveraging the vagus nerve's power to resist inflammation.

- Elevate Mood and Mental Clarity: Harness the vagus nerve's potential to enhance mood, eliminate brain fog, and support mental well-being.

- Restore Balance: Achieve a harmonious harmony in your body and mind by engaging the vagus nerve's intrinsic capacity for self-regulation.

- Heal from Within: Explore innovative self-healing techniques and practices that tap into the vagus nerve's remarkable potential.

Packed with concrete insights, practical exercises, and the latest scientific data, the "Vagus Nerve Gut Wonder Handbook" is your entire guide to a healthier, happier life. Whether you seek relief from stress, digestive woes, or a profound sense of inner serenity, this book provides the keys to unlock your body's hidden treasure — the vagus nerve.

Prepare to embark on a transforming trip as you delve into the mystical world of your vagus nerve. Are you ready to reinvent your health story and enjoy a life of wonder, balance, and vitality? If the answer is yes, then this manual is your important companion on the path to wellness.

Join the thousands who have already awakened the vagus nerve's immense potential and embark on a journey toward a healthier, more peaceful life. The Vagus Nerve

Gut Wonder Handbook is your key to a new dimension of well-being. Get your copy today and start experiencing the wonder within!

CHAPTER ONE

ANATOMY AND FUNCTION OF THE VAGUS NERVE

The vagus nerve, often referred to as the "wanderer" or "vagabond" nerve, is one of the most intriguing and essential components of the human nervous system. This cranial nerve, known as the tenth cranial nerve (CN X), possesses an intricate anatomy and a wide array of functions that extend far beyond the boundaries of traditional neurology. In this book, we will embark on an enlightening journey through the intricate world of the vagus nerve, exploring its anatomy, functions, and profound influence on our physical, mental, and emotional well-being.

Anatomy of the Vagus Nerve

The vagus nerve is a bilateral pair of cranial nerves that extend from the brain-stem through the neck and into the chest and abdomen. It is aptly named for its extensive distribution, as "vagus" is derived from the Latin word for "wandering." This nerve is comprised of both sensory and motor fibres, making it a versatile and multifunctional component of the autonomic nervous system (ANS).

The vagus nerve originates in the medulla oblongata, the lowest part of the brainstem. It emerges from the brain as two separate nuclei, the dorsal motor nucleus and the nucleus ambiguus, which give rise to the motor fibers responsible for controlling various visceral functions. As the vagus nerve descends through the neck, it branches out into multiple fibers, with the left and right vagus nerves ultimately connecting to organs and tissues throughout the body.

Notably, the vagus nerve has both afferent (sensory) and efferent (motor) components. The afferent fibers relay sensory information from visceral organs to the brain, providing crucial feedback on the body's internal state. In contrast, the efferent fibers carry signals from the brain to organs, regulating processes such as digestion, heart rate, and respiration.

Functions of the Vagus Nerve

The vagus nerve is involved in a vast array of physiological processes, and its functions can be categorized into the following key areas:

Parasympathetic Nervous System Control: The vagus nerve plays a central role in the parasympathetic nervous system (PNS), often referred to as the "rest and digest" system. It regulates bodily functions during times of rest and recovery, including slowing the heart rate, promoting digestion, and conserving energy.

Cardiovascular Regulation: The vagus nerve exerts control over the heart rate and rhythm, helping to maintain cardiovascular stability. It can slow down the heart rate in response to relaxation and facilitate rapid adjustments in response to stress.

Gastrointestinal Function: This nerve is a key player in digestive processes, controlling the release of digestive enzymes, peristalsis, and nutrient absorption. It also conveys signals of fullness and satisfaction to the brain.

Inflammatory Response: The vagus nerve has a remarkable anti-inflammatory effect on the body. It can dampen excessive inflammation by signaling the release of anti-inflammatory molecules, thus playing a pivotal role in the body's immune response.

Respiratory Control: The vagus nerve regulates breathing, influencing both the rate and depth of respiration. It is involved in reflexes such as coughing, swallowing, and sneezing.

Emotional and Psychological Well-being: Emerging research suggests that the vagus nerve is intricately linked to emotional and mental health. It plays a role in mood regulation, anxiety reduction, and may even contribute to conditions like depression when dysfunction occurs.

Social Engagement: The vagus nerve is associated with the body's social engagement system. It enables facial expressions, vocalizations, and gestures that facilitate communication and connection with others.

CHAPTER TWO

THE GUT-BRAIN AXIS

The gut-brain connection, commonly referred to as the "second brain," is a fascinating and intricate interaction between your digestive system and your central neurological system. It's a dynamic, bidirectional communication system that continuously trades information, substantially altering your physical and emotional well-being.

At the center of this connection lies the vagus nerve, a neurological superhighway between your gut and brain. This conduit permits your gut to convey messages to your brain, influencing your mood, emotions, and even decision-making. Conversely, your brain communicates with your gut, impacting digestive processes and general gut health.

This delicate interplay isn't confined to the vagus nerve; it also involves a complex network of neurons, hormones, and neurotransmitters. The gut houses millions of neurons, sometimes referred to as the "enteric nervous system," which may work autonomously, earning its reputation as the "second brain." This "brain" orchestrates the digestive process, making decisions and modifications without conscious thought.

The gut-brain link isn't just about digesting; it deeply effects your mental health. Research has demonstrated that imbalances in gut flora, known as the microbiome, might influence mood disorders like anxiety and depression. Moreover, your gut creates neurotransmitters like serotonin, a critical factor in controlling mood.

Understanding the gut-brain link empowers us to make informed lifestyle choices. A balanced diet, high in fiber and probiotics, supports gut health and, in turn, positively influences your mood and cognitive function. Stress management approaches like mindfulness and meditation can help increase this connection, as persistent stress can break it.

In essence, the gut-brain link is a testament to the holistic nature of our bodies. It highlights the need of preserving not just bodily but also mental well-being. By nourishing your gut and regulating stress, you may harness the power of this unique partnership for a happier, healthier life.

COMMUNICATION PATHWAYS BETWEEN THE GUT AND BRAIN

The communication pathways between the gut and the brain are a remarkable aspect of our body's functioning. While we often think of these two organs as distinct entities, they are intricately connected through a complex network of nerves and biochemical signals.

The primary link in this connection is the vagus nerve, which acts as a bi-directional highway between the gut and the brain. This nerve relays information from the gut to the brain and vice versa. For example, when you eat, sensory information about the food's composition and digestion progress is sent to the brain via the vagus nerve. In response, the brain can then send signals back to the gut, influencing processes like digestion and appetite.

Beyond the vagus nerve, various biochemical messengers, such as hormones and neurotransmitters, play a crucial role in this gut-brain dialogue. For instance, the gut produces serotonin, a neurotransmitter that affects mood and well-being. This highlights the "gut feeling" we sometimes experience in emotionally charged situations.

This intricate communication pathway isn't limited to just physical processes. Research suggests it also has a significant impact on our emotions and mental health. Conditions like stress, anxiety, and depression can influence gut function, and conversely, an imbalanced gut can affect our mood.

Understanding the communication pathways between the gut and the brain underscores the importance of a holistic approach to health. It reminds us that taking care of our gut through a balanced diet, regular exercise, and stress management isn't just about physical well-being — it's also about nurturing our emotional and mental health. This bidirectional conversation between our gut and brain is a fascinating aspect of our body's design, revealing the intricate connections that contribute to our overall wellness.

HOW EMOTIONS IMPACT GUT HEALTH

Emotions and gut health share a profound connection that often goes unnoticed in our daily lives. The human body is a complex tapestry of interwoven systems, and the influence of our emotions on the gut is a prime example of this intricate relationship.

When we experience strong emotions like stress, anxiety, or sadness, it's not just our minds that are affected. These emotions can send signals to our gut, triggering physical reactions. This connection is often referred to as the "gut-brain axis."

For instance, when we're stressed, our body's "fight or flight" response kicks in. This response, controlled by the autonomic nervous system, can divert blood flow away from the digestive system, leading to issues like indigestion or an upset stomach. Chronic stress can also disrupt the balance of gut bacteria, potentially leading to more serious digestive problems in the long term.

On the flip side, a healthy gut can positively influence our emotional well-being. The gut is home to millions of micro-organisms, collectively known as the gut microbiota. These microbes play a crucial role in digesting food and producing essential nutrients. Recent research has shown that they also communicate with the brain, influencing our mood and emotions. A balanced gut microbiome is thought to contribute to better mental health and emotional stability.

So, it's a two-way street: our emotions can impact our gut health, and the state of our gut can influence our emotions. It's a reminder that caring for our emotional well-being isn't just about what happens in our minds but extends to how our bodies respond, especially in the gut. Nurturing a healthy gut through a balanced diet, regular exercise, and stress management can, in turn, help us better manage our emotions and lead to overall improved well-being. This intricate connection between our emotions and gut health underscores the importance of a holistic approach to health and self-care.

CHAPTER THREE

VAGUS NERVE DYSFUNCTION

The vagus nerve, a crucial part of our autonomic nervous system, is responsible for regulating many vital functions in our body. When it doesn't work as it should, it can lead to a condition known as vagus nerve dysfunction.

This dysfunction can manifest in various ways, affecting digestion, heart rate, and even our emotional well-being. People with vagus nerve dysfunction may experience symptoms like heart palpitations, digestive problems, anxiety, and difficulty in managing stress.

Understanding and addressing vagus nerve dysfunction is vital because it can impact our overall health and quality of life. Lifestyle changes, stress management techniques, and sometimes medical interventions can help restore balance and improve symptoms associated with this condition.

If you suspect you may have vagus nerve dysfunction, it's essential to consult with a healthcare professional who can provide a proper diagnosis and guidance on the most appropriate treatment options for your specific situation.

SIGNS AND SYMPTOMS OF A DYSFUNCTIONAL VAGUS NERVE

A dysfunctional vagus nerve, can manifest through various signs and symptoms, often impacting our overall well-being. Here's a summary of what to look out for:

Digestive Issues: You may experience frequent stomach problems, such as bloating, constipation, or diarrhoea. These issues can be a result of impaired digestive regulation by the vagus nerve.

Heart Rate Irregularities: A vagus nerve dysfunction can lead to heart rate irregularities. You might notice an elevated or erratic heart rate even during non-stressful situations.

Chronic Fatigue: A tired feeling that doesn't improve with rest is common. The vagus nerve helps regulate energy levels, and dysfunction can lead to persistent fatigue.

Anxiety and Mood Swings: Emotional instability, anxiety, and mood swings may occur. The vagus nerve influences emotional regulation, and disruptions can affect your mental well-being.

Breathing Problems: Shallow or irregular breathing patterns might develop. The vagus nerve controls respiration, so dysfunction can affect your ability to breathe deeply and calmly.

Poor Immune Response: Frequent illnesses or slow recovery from infections may indicate a compromised vagus nerve. It plays a role in modulating the immune system.

Chronic Inflammation: Excessive inflammation in the body may result from vagus nerve dysfunction. This can contribute to various health issues.

Difficulty Swallowing: You might have trouble swallowing or a sensation of a lump in your throat. These issues can be linked to impaired vagal function.

Speech and Voice Changes: Changes in your voice, such as hoarseness or difficulty speaking clearly, can also be associated with vagus nerve dysfunction.

Dizziness and Fainting: Feeling light-headed, dizzy, or experiencing fainting spells may occur due to blood pressure and heart rate fluctuations controlled by the vagus nerve.

If you suspect vagus nerve dysfunction based on these signs, consulting a healthcare professional is essential. They can provide a proper diagnosis and recommend treatments or lifestyle changes to help restore vagus nerve function and improve your overall health and well-being.

FACTORS CONTRIBUTING TO VAGUS NERVE DYSFUNCTION

Vagus Nerve Dysfunction, often overlooked but increasingly recognized, can be attributed to various factors:

Chronic Stress: Prolonged stress can overstimulate the sympathetic nervous system and inhibit the vagus nerve's calming influence, leading to dysfunction.

Inflammatory Conditions: Conditions like autoimmune disorders, infections, or chronic inflammation can disrupt vagal function.

Digestive Issues: Gut problems, such as irritable bowel syndrome (IBS) or gastrointestinal disorders, may impact the vagus nerve's role in digestion.

Physical Trauma: Injuries to the head, neck, or chest can damage the vagus nerve or impede its signals.

Sedentary Lifestyle: Lack of physical activity can affect overall nerve function, including the vagus nerve.

Poor Diet: Unhealthy eating habits, especially diets high in processed foods, can lead to gut imbalances that affect the vagus nerve.

Certain Medications: Some medications, such as beta-blockers, can interfere with vagus nerve activity.

Psychological Factors: Conditions like anxiety, depression, or post-traumatic stress disorder (PTSD) may contribute to vagus nerve dysfunction.

Excessive Alcohol or Tobacco Use: Substance abuse can impair nerve function, including the vagus nerve.

Chronic Illness: Conditions like diabetes or heart disease can indirectly impact vagal function due to their effects on the body.

It's essential to recognize these contributing factors and address them in managing Vagus Nerve Dysfunction for better overall health and well-being.

CHAPTER FOUR

TECHNIQUES TO HEAL AND STRENGTHEN THE VAGUS NERVE

A weakened or impaired vagus nerve can lead to a host of health issues, both physical and mental. Fortunately, there are ways to heal and strengthen this vital nerve, offering a pathway to enhanced overall well-being.

Deep Breathing

One of the most accessible and effective ways to stimulate the vagus nerve is through deep, diaphragmatic breathing. Slow, intentional breaths, where you fill your abdomen rather than shallowly breathing into your chest, can trigger the relaxation response mediated by the vagus nerve. This practice helps reduce stress, anxiety, and even lowers blood pressure.

Cold Exposure

Exposing yourself to cold, such as taking cold showers or immersing yourself in cold water (cryotherapy), can stimulate the vagus nerve. The body's response to cold includes an increase in heart rate, followed by a subsequent drop, and this process can activate the vagus nerve, promoting overall cardiovascular health.

Yoga and Meditation

Mind-body practices like yoga and meditation have long been recognized for their vagus nerve-stimulating effects. These practices encourage relaxation, deep breathing, and mindfulness, all of which can engage and strengthen the vagus nerve. Regular sessions can contribute to reduced stress and improved emotional well-being.

Laughter and Social Connection

Laughter truly is the best medicine, and it can also be a tonic for the vagus nerve. Genuine laughter and positive social interactions stimulate the vagus nerve, triggering the release of beneficial neurochemicals that promote a sense of happiness and overall emotional balance. Surrounding yourself with loved ones and engaging in activities that make you laugh can be a simple yet potent remedy.

Gargling and Singing

Surprisingly, the simple act of gargling or singing loudly can stimulate the vagus nerve, as these activities involve the muscles in the back of the throat that are connected to the nerve. Singing, in particular, not only engages the vagus nerve but also releases endorphins, providing a dual benefit for emotional well-being.

Probiotics and Gut Health

The gut-brain connection is intimately linked to the vagus nerve. A healthy gut microbiome, maintained through the consumption of probiotics and a fiber-rich diet, can positively influence vagal tone, which is essential for maintaining gut health and emotional balance.

In our quest for well-being, the vagus nerve occupies a central role, orchestrating a symphony of bodily functions. By incorporating these techniques into our daily lives, we have the power to heal and strengthen this remarkable nerve, fostering not only physical health but also emotional balance. In doing so, we tap into our body's innate capacity for self-regulation and well-being, unlocking the potential for a healthier, more vibrant life.

NUTRITIONAL APPROACHES TO SUPPORT VAGUS NERVE HEALING

But what if our vagus nerve is out of tune? The good news is that through mindful nutritional choices, we can support its healing and optimize its functioning. Let's embark on a journey into the realm of nutritional approaches to nurture and rejuvenate this incredible nerve.

1. Omega-3 Fatty Acids:

Found abundantly in fatty fish like salmon, mackerel, and flaxseeds, omega-3 fatty acids are renowned for their anti-inflammatory properties. Inflammation can impede the vagus nerve's ability to transmit signals effectively. By incorporating these healthy fats into our diet, we provide the raw materials needed for nerve repair and help reduce inflammation, promoting vagal tone.

2. Leafy Greens and Antioxidants:

The vagus nerve dances to the rhythm of our autonomic nervous system, and oxidative stress can disrupt this delicate balance. To counteract this, fill your plate with antioxidant-rich foods like kale, spinach, and berries. These gems not only combat oxidative stress but also nurture a thriving environment for your vagus nerve to flourish.

3. Probiotics and Gut Health:

Did you know that a significant portion of your vagus nerve's connections reside in your gut? A flourishing microbiome is essential for a healthy vagus nerve. Fermented foods like yogurt, kefir, and kimchi are brimming with probiotics, which can enhance gut health and consequently support the vagus nerve's functions.

4. Mindful Eating and the Gut-Brain Connection:

The act of mindful eating isn't just a trendy practice; it's a direct path to vagal healing. Slow down, savor your meals, and be present with your food. This practice engages the parasympathetic nervous system (which the vagus nerve is a part of), promoting relaxation and optimal digestion.

5. Herbal Allies:

Certain herbs have a long history of supporting nervous system health. Chamomile, lavender, and lemon balm are known for their calming effects, reducing stress and anxiety that can negatively impact the vagus nerve. Enjoy them as teas or incorporate them into your meals.

6. Reduce Sugar and Processed Foods:

Excessive sugar and processed foods can wreak havoc on our gut health and, by extension, our vagus nerve.

Cutting back on these culprits can prevent inflammation and ensure the nerve's smooth operation.

Nurturing the vagus nerve through nutritional approaches is a profound act of self-care. It's about recognizing the intimate connection between what we eat and how we feel, both physically and emotionally. As we make conscious choices to support our vagus nerve, we embark on a path toward greater well-being and inner harmony, where the "wanderer" nerve can find its true north once more.

PHYSICAL ACTIVITY AND ITS ROLE IN VAGUS NERVE HEALTH

The vagus nerve has two main branches: sensory (afferent) and motor (efferent) fibers. The sensory fibers transmit information from our internal organs to the brain, providing vital feedback about our body's condition.

Meanwhile, the motor fibers convey signals from the brain to our organs, regulating various physiological processes.

Now, let's explore the connection between physical activity and the health of the vagus nerve.

Heart Rate Regulation: One of the most well-known functions of the vagus nerve is its influence on heart rate. When at rest, a healthy vagus nerve helps slow down our heart rate, promoting relaxation. Regular physical activity, such as aerobic exercise, challenges the vagus nerve in a positive way. As we engage in exercise, the heart rate increases, providing the vagus nerve with opportunities for stimulation and adaptation. Over time, this can contribute to improved heart rate variability, a marker of overall heart health.

Stress Reduction: Physical activity has a well-documented ability to reduce stress levels. When we exercise, the vagus nerve plays a role in dampening the body's "fight or flight" response and shifting it towards the "rest and digest" mode. This shift can lead to reduced stress hormones like cortisol and increased feelings of relaxation, all of which contribute to vagal nerve health.

Digestive Health: The vagus nerve also influences digestion by regulating the release of digestive enzymes and promoting peristalsis, the rhythmic contractions of the digestive tract. Regular physical activity can enhance these processes, aiding in better digestion and absorption of nutrients.

Inflammation Control: Emerging research suggests that physical activity may help reduce inflammation in the body, partly due to its impact on the vagus nerve. When the vagus nerve is activated, it can signal the release of anti-inflammatory molecules, potentially playing a role in mitigating chronic inflammation.

Mood and Mental Well-being: Physical activity has a profound impact on mood and mental health. Some studies indicate that exercise can stimulate the vagus nerve, leading to mood improvements and potentially offering therapeutic benefits for conditions like depression and anxiety.

Understanding the relationship between physical activity and vagus nerve health sheds light on the importance of an active lifestyle in maintaining overall well-being. Engaging in regular exercise not only enhances physical fitness but also contributes to the harmonious functioning of the vagus nerve, promoting better heart health, stress resilience, digestion, and potentially even mental and emotional balance. As we continue to explore the intricate web of connections within our bodies, it becomes increasingly clear that the road to holistic health often begins with something as simple as taking a walk or engaging in your favorite physical activity.

CHAPTER FIVE

DIET AND NUTRITION FOR A HEALTHY GUT

Imagine, if you will, an entire universe residing within your digestive tract. This is the gut microbiome: a vast community of micro-organisms that includes bacteria, viruses, fungi, and more. These microscopic beings, numbering in the trillions, form a complex web of interactions that can influence virtually every aspect of your well-being.

The Diversity of Life

Diversity is the hallmark of a thriving ecosystem, and the gut microbiome is no exception. In this microscopic realm, a wide array of microbial species coexists, each with its own specialized role to play. Some are beneficial, aiding in digestion and nutrient absorption, while others are opportunistic pathogens that, when kept in check, pose no harm.

A Balancing Act

Maintaining a delicate balance among these diverse inhabitants is critical. A shift in this equilibrium, known as dysbiosis, can have profound consequences for your health. It can lead to digestive disorders, immune system dysfunction, and even impact your mental well-being. The importance of this equilibrium cannot be overstated.

Health Implications

The gut microbiome isn't just a passive bystander; it actively participates in various bodily processes. It's deeply involved in digestion, breaking down complex carbohydrates and producing essential vitamins and nutrients. Moreover, it plays a pivotal role in the development and functioning of the immune system, acting as a defense force against invading pathogens.

Recent research has uncovered the gut microbiome's impact on our mental health, with the gut-brain axis emerging as a hot topic. It seems that the trillions of microbes in our gut can communicate with our brain, influencing mood, behavior, and potentially contributing to conditions like anxiety and depression.

A Tale of Diet and Lifestyle

Your daily choices hold immense sway over the health of your gut microbiome. Diet, in particular, is a powerful determinant. Consuming a diverse range of fiber-rich foods, such as fruits, vegetables, and whole grains, promotes the growth of beneficial microbes. In contrast, a diet high in sugar and processed foods can fuel the growth of less desirable micro-organisms.

Lifestyle factors, too, come into play. Stress, sleep, and physical activity can all impact the composition and functioning of your gut microbiome. A harmonious life is reflected in a harmonious microbiome.

The Power of Probiotics and Prebiotics

Harnessing the potential of the gut microbiome for health benefits has given rise to the popularity of probiotics and prebiotics. Probiotics are live beneficial bacteria found in certain foods and supplements, while prebiotics are the non-digestible fibers that nourish these helpful microbes. Together, they can aid in restoring and maintaining a balanced gut microbiome.

The gut microbiome is nothing short of a fascinating ecosystem—a universe within us that impacts our physical, mental, and emotional health. As science delves deeper into this microscopic world, we gain a greater understanding of how to nurture and preserve its delicate balance. It's a testament to the intricate wonders of the human body and a reminder that our health is intimately linked to the microscopic life forms within us. So, let us cherish and care for this thriving ecosystem, for in its health lies the foundation of our own.

FOODS THAT NOURISH THE GUT-BRAIN AXIS

The foods we consume play a pivotal role in shaping this intricate connection, influencing not only our digestive health but also our mental and emotional well-being.

1. Probiotic-Rich Fermented Foods: The Gut's Best Friends

Fermented foods like yoghurt, kefir, sauerkraut, and kimchi are teeming with beneficial bacteria known as probiotics. These micro-organisms, such as Lactobacillus and Bifidobacterium strains, colonize the gut and contribute to its microbial diversity. A flourishing gut microbiome is essential for a balanced gut-brain axis. Probiotics support digestion, fortify the intestinal lining, and even manufacture neurotransmitters like serotonin. These "feel-good" molecules are vital for mood regulation and can significantly impact mental health. Ingesting probiotic-rich foods is like cultivating a lush garden in your gut, fostering harmony between your mind and your digestive system.

2. Prebiotic-Rich Fiber: Fertilizing Your Microbial Garden

Prebiotics are indigestible fibers found in foods like chicory root, garlic, onions, and artichokes. They serve as nourishment for the probiotics in your gut, promoting their growth and activity. By incorporating prebiotic-rich foods into your diet, you provide your gut bacteria with the sustenance they need to thrive.

This microbial "feast" leads to the production of short-chain fatty acids (SCFAs), such as butyrate. SCFAs are like messengers that travel from the gut to the brain, influencing cognitive function and mood regulation. A diet rich in prebiotic fibers not only supports digestion but also nurtures a positive gut-brain connection.

3. Omega-3 Fatty Acids: Brain Food from the Sea

Fatty fish like salmon, mackerel, and sardines are abundant sources of omega-3 fatty acids. These essential fats, particularly eicosapentaenoic acid (EPA) and docosahexaenoic acid (DHA), are renowned for their brain-boosting properties.

Omega-3s not only reduce inflammation in the gut but also support a healthy gut lining. They assist in the production of anti-inflammatory molecules, which can modulate the gut-brain axis by quelling excessive inflammation that may contribute to mood disorders.

4. Polyphenol-Packed Plant Foods: Guardians of Cognitive Health

Polyphenols, found in foods like berries, dark chocolate, and green tea, are potent antioxidants with neuro-protective properties. They combat oxidative stress and inflammation, shielding both the gut and the brain from harm.

These compounds can influence the gut-brain axis by enhancing the diversity of gut bacteria and promoting the growth of beneficial strains. Furthermore, polyphenols may stimulate the release of brain-derived neurotrophic factor (BDNF), a protein essential for cognitive function and mood regulation.

5. Complex Carbohydrates: Fuel for Brain and Gut

Whole grains, legumes, and starchy vegetables provide a steady supply of complex carbohydrates. These foods offer a sustained release of energy, stabilizing blood sugar levels and fostering a sense of well-being.

Complex carbs also promote the growth of Bifidobacteria in the gut, which can contribute to the production of neurotransmitters like serotonin. This dual benefit supports both digestive health and emotional equilibrium.

The relationship between the gut and the brain is an intricate dance orchestrated by the foods we choose to consume. By embracing a diet rich in probiotics, prebiotics, omega-3 fatty acids, polyphenols, and complex carbohydrates, we nourish this connection, enhancing both our physical and mental vitality. The gut-brain axis, when properly tended to through mindful nutrition, becomes a harmonious duet that resonates with overall well-being and contentment. In the world of human biology, it's a symphony worth savoring.

PROBIOTICS, PREBIOTICS, AND GUT-HEALTHY RECIPES

Our journey into the world of gut health begins with two essential terms: probiotics and prebiotics. These words have been buzzing in health circles for some time, but what do they really mean, and why are they crucial for our well-being? This guide aims to unravel the mysteries of these gut superheroes and provide you with delectable, gut-nourishing recipes to kickstart your journey to a healthier you.

Probiotics: The Gut's Best Friends

Probiotics are live micro-organisms, commonly referred to as "good bacteria," that provide a multitude of benefits when ingested. These beneficial bacteria take residence in our gastrointestinal tract, helping to maintain a balanced and thriving gut microbiome. They play a pivotal role in digestion, nutrient absorption, and immune system support. Some common sources of probiotics include yogurt, kefir, sauerkraut, kimchi, and certain supplements.

But it's not just about the what; it's also about the why. Probiotics can help:

Digestion: Probiotics assist in breaking down food and absorbing essential nutrients, aiding in more efficient digestion.

Immunity: A robust gut microbiome contributes to a resilient immune system, helping to ward off infections and illnesses.

Mood: Emerging research suggests a gut-brain connection. A balanced gut can positively impact mood and reduce the risk of anxiety and depression.

Skin Health: A well-balanced gut microbiome can lead to clearer, healthier skin by reducing inflammation and promoting nutrient absorption.

Prebiotics: The Food for Good Bacteria

Prebiotics, often less known but equally important, are non-digestible fibers found in certain foods. They act as food for the probiotics, promoting their growth and activity in the gut. Sources of prebiotics include garlic, onions, leeks, asparagus, and bananas.

Prebiotics are essential because they:

Feed Probiotics: Prebiotics serve as sustenance for the good bacteria, allowing them to thrive and multiply.

Support Digestion: By promoting the growth of beneficial bacteria, prebiotics contribute to a healthy gut environment and smooth digestion.

Balance Gut Flora: Prebiotics help maintain the balance between good and bad bacteria, fostering a harmonious gut ecosystem.

A healthy gut isn't just about digestion; it's about overall well-being. Welcome to a culinary adventure that combines the pleasures of gastronomy with the benefits of gut health. In this collection, we'll explore 30 diverse, flavorful, and nutrient-rich recipes that not only tantalize your taste buds but also nourish your gut.

Breakfast Delights

Creamy Greek Yoghurt Parfait: Start your day with a probiotic-rich treat topped with fresh berries and honey.

Overnight Oats with Chia Seeds: A fiber-packed breakfast that supports a balanced gut microbiome.

Avocado and Spinach Breakfast Wrap: A savory and fiber-filled way to kick-start your morning.

Soup for the Soul

Roasted Butternut Squash Soup: A velvety blend of flavors with gut-soothing properties.

Miso Soup: Packed with probiotics, this Japanese classic promotes a healthy gut.

Hearty Lentil Stew: A high-fiber, plant-based stew that nourishes both body and soul.

Vibrant Salads

Kale and Quinoa Salad: A nutrient-dense salad loaded with fiber and antioxidants.

Fermented Kimchi Salad: Probiotic-rich kimchi adds a flavorful twist to this crunchy medley.

Colorful Beet and Carrot Slaw: A rainbow of vegetables for a diverse gut microbiome.

Savory Mains

Baked Salmon with Lemon and Dill: Omega-3 fatty acids support gut health and reduce inflammation.

Chickpea and Sweet Potato Curry: A delightful blend of spices and legumes for digestive harmony.

Grilled Portobello Mushrooms: A savory and fiber-packed alternative for meat lovers.

Satisfying Sides

Garlic and Herb Roasted Broccoli: Fiber and prebiotics combine for gut-friendly goodness.

Turmeric-Cauliflower Rice: Anti-inflammatory turmeric adds depth to this low-carb side.

Sautéed Spinach with Garlic: A simple, nutrient-rich side dish that supports gut health.

Snacktime Pleasures

Homemade Hummus with Veggies: Fiber-rich chickpeas and a rainbow of crunchy dippers.

Trail Mix with Nuts and Dried Fruit: A perfect balance of fiber, protein, and healthy fats.

Gut-Friendly Smoothie: A blend of kefir, banana, and berries for a probiotic punch.

Sweet Treats

Dark Chocolate and Berry Parfait: A guilt-free dessert packed with antioxidants.

Banana Nut Muffins: A comforting, high-fiber snack for those with a sweet tooth.

Chia Seed Pudding with Berries: A delightful dessert loaded with fiber and omega-3s.

Fermented Favorites

Homemade Kombucha: Brew your gut-loving probiotic elixir.

Sauerkraut: A simple and tangy side dish that's also a probiotic powerhouse.

Yoghurt and Berry Smoothie Bowl: A visually stunning breakfast filled with gut-friendly ingredients.

Artisanal Breads and Spreads

Whole Grain Sourdough Bread: A rustic loaf that's easier on the gut than conventional bread.

Cashew Nut Butter: Creamy, homemade nut butter for a dose of healthy fats.

Zucchini Bread: A delicious and moist loaf that incorporates gut-loving veggies.

With these 30 gut-healthy recipes, you have the tools to embark on a culinary journey that not only tantalizes your palate but also nurtures your gut. Remember, a balanced gut contributes to overall well-being, so savor each dish, share them with loved ones, and relish the joy of nourishing your body from the inside out. Happy cooking, and here's to a healthier, happier you!

CHAPTER SIX

STRESS REDUCTION AND RELAXATION

When stress strikes, a series of physiological reactions is set in motion. The "fight or flight" response, designed for immediate survival, activates. Hormones like cortisol and adrenaline surge through the bloodstream, preparing the body for action. But what happens when stress becomes chronic, when it lingers like an unwelcome guest?

The gut, it seems, has a story to tell in this narrative. Researchers have discovered that the gut and the brain engage in an intricate dialogue via the gut-brain axis. This bi-directional communication system comprises neural, hormonal, and immunological pathways that enable the two to exchange vital information. When stress persists, the gut-brain axis can become dysregulated. This dysregulation can have far-reaching consequences.

The gut microbiome, once harmonious and balanced, can undergo significant shifts. Beneficial bacteria may dwindle, allowing opportunistic pathogens to flourish. This imbalance, known as dysbiosis, can lead to a cascade of health issues. Digestive disturbances, immune dysfunction, and even mood disorders can arise as the gut microbiome's equilibrium is disrupted.

But the gut's woes do not end there. It appears that this microbial community can influence our response to stress as well. Recent studies have unveiled that a healthy gut microbiome can foster resilience to stress, helping individuals cope better with life's challenges. Conversely, a disrupted microbiome may contribute to heightened stress sensitivity.

While the stress-gut connection holds intrigue, it also presents opportunities for intervention. Lifestyle modifications, such as dietary changes and stress management techniques, can positively impact the gut microbiome. Incorporating probiotics and prebiotics into one's diet may help restore balance to the gut's microcosm. Additionally, mindfulness practices and relaxation techniques can serve as antidotes to chronic stress, thereby supporting a healthier gut-brain axis.

The stress-gut connection is a captivating tale of two worlds converging in our bodies. It reminds us that our emotional well-being is intimately entwined with our physical health. As we unravel the intricacies of this connection, we discover not only the vulnerability of our internal metropolis but also its resilience. By nurturing our gut, we can foster a harmony between our emotional and physical selves, ultimately leading to a richer and more balanced existence.

TECHNIQUES FOR MANAGING STRESS AND ANXIETY

Stress and anxiety are common experiences in today's fast-paced world, affecting people of all ages and backgrounds. While they are natural responses to challenging situations, chronic stress and anxiety can have detrimental effects on physical and mental well-being. Fortunately, there are several effective techniques to manage and reduce stress and anxiety. Here, we will explore some of these techniques in detail.

Deep Breathing Exercises: Deep breathing is a simple yet powerful technique that can help calm the nervous system and reduce stress. Practicing deep breathing involves taking slow, deep breaths in through the nose, holding for a few seconds, and exhaling slowly through the mouth. This technique can be done anywhere and is particularly effective in the midst of a stressful situation.

Progressive Muscle Relaxation: This technique involves systematically tensing and then relaxing different muscle groups in the body. By doing this, it can help release physical tension associated with stress and promote a sense of relaxation. Regular practice can lead to improved body awareness and reduced overall tension.

Mindfulness Meditation: Mindfulness meditation involves focusing on the present moment without judgement. By observing thoughts, emotions, and sensations without trying to change them, individuals can develop greater awareness and acceptance. Numerous studies have shown that mindfulness meditation can significantly reduce symptoms of anxiety and stress.

Regular Exercise: Physical activity is a powerful stress reducer. Engaging in regular exercise releases endorphins, which are natural mood lifters. Exercise also helps improve sleep quality, increase energy levels, and reduce muscle tension—all of which can contribute to lower stress and anxiety.

Healthy Lifestyle Choices: Proper nutrition and adequate sleep play crucial roles in managing stress and anxiety. A well-balanced diet rich in whole foods and adequate sleep (typically 7-9 hours per night) can improve resilience to stress and promote emotional well-being.

Social Support: Connecting with friends and loved ones can provide a significant emotional buffer against stress and anxiety. Sharing feelings and concerns with trusted individuals can be comforting and provide valuable perspectives and advice.

Time Management: Effective time management can reduce the feeling of being overwhelmed by tasks and responsibilities. Prioritizing tasks, setting realistic goals, and breaking tasks into smaller, manageable steps can all help alleviate stress associated with a busy schedule.

Limiting Stimulants: Reducing the intake of stimulants like caffeine and nicotine can have a positive impact on anxiety levels. These substances can exacerbate feelings of nervousness and restlessness.

Therapy and Counseling: For individuals dealing with chronic or severe anxiety, seeking the help of a mental health professional can be highly beneficial. Cognitive-behavioral therapy (CBT) and other therapeutic approaches can teach coping strategies and provide valuable support.

Self-Care: Taking time for self-care activities that bring joy and relaxation can be an effective way to manage stress and anxiety. This can include hobbies, leisure activities, or spending time in nature.

It's important to note that what works best can vary from person to person. A combination of these techniques may be most effective for some individuals. It's also crucial to remember that seeking professional help is a valid and valuable option if stress and anxiety become overwhelming or persistent. With commitment and practice, these techniques can empower individuals to take control of their stress and anxiety, leading to a more balanced and fulfilling life.

CREATING A RELAXATION ROUTINE FOR VAGUS NERVE HEALTH

The vagus nerve is a crucial part of the autonomic nervous system, responsible for regulating various bodily functions, including heart rate, digestion, and stress response. Maintaining the health of your vagus nerve can have a profound impact on your overall well-being, as it plays a significant role in reducing stress, inflammation, and improving overall mental and physical health. Establishing a relaxation routine to support vagus nerve health is a valuable practice that can enhance your quality of life. Here's a brief yet detailed guide on how to create such a routine:

Deep Breathing:

Begin your relaxation routine with deep, diaphragmatic breathing. Sit or lie down comfortably, close your eyes, and take slow, deep breaths.

Inhale deeply through your nose for a count of four, allowing your abdomen to rise as you fill your lungs.

Exhale slowly through your mouth for a count of six, focusing on completely emptying your lungs.

Repeat this deep breathing pattern for 3-5 minutes. Deep breathing stimulates the vagus nerve, promoting relaxation and reducing stress.

Meditation:

Incorporate meditation into your routine. Find a quiet space and sit or lie down comfortably.

Focus your attention on your breath or use a guided meditation app or recording.

Engaging in mindfulness meditation can activate the vagus nerve and help lower stress levels.

Progressive Muscle Relaxation:

Tense and release various muscle groups in your body. Start from your toes and work your way up to your head. Hold each muscle group tensed for a few seconds and then release. Pay attention to the sensation of relaxation as you release tension.

This technique can help reduce muscle tension and promote relaxation, stimulating the vagus nerve.

Yoga:

Practice yoga postures and stretches that emphasize deep breathing and relaxation, such as child's pose, corpse pose (savasana), and the bridge pose.

Yoga combines physical movement with controlled breathing, which can activate the vagus nerve and reduce stress.

Social Engagement:

Engage in activities that promote social connection, like spending time with loved ones, joining clubs or groups, or volunteering.

Positive social interactions can stimulate the vagus nerve, as it is closely tied to our social engagement system.

Cold Exposure:

End your relaxation routine with a cold exposure element, such as a cold shower or a brief cold-water immersion. Cold exposure can activate the vagus nerve, improve circulation, and enhance overall nervous system function.

Regularity:

Consistency is key. Aim to incorporate your relaxation routine into your daily or weekly schedule.

Regular practice can strengthen the vagus nerve's responsiveness over time, leading to long-term benefits for your well-being.

Incorporating these practices into your life can help create a relaxation routine that supports vagus nerve health. Remember that it may take time to experience noticeable benefits, so be patient and persistent in your efforts. Prioritizing your vagus nerve health can have a positive impact on your overall physical and mental well-being, helping you better manage stress and maintain a state of relaxation in your daily life.

CHAPTER SEVEN

SLEEP AND GUT HEALTH

Sleep is a fundamental aspect of human health and well-being. It plays a crucial role in physical and mental restoration, cognitive function, and overall quality of life. Unfortunately, many individuals struggle with sleep-related issues, such as insomnia or poor sleep quality. Here, we explore effective strategies to enhance sleep quality naturally, without resorting to medication or other artificial aids.

Maintain a Consistent Sleep Schedule:

Try to go to bed and wake up at the same time every day, even on weekends. This helps regulate your body's internal clock, making it easier to fall asleep and wake up refreshed.

Create a Relaxing Bedtime Routine:

Establishing a calming pre-sleep routine can signal to your body that it's time to wind down. Activities like reading, gentle stretching, or taking a warm bath can prepare your mind and body for sleep.

Optimize Your Sleep Environment:

Make your bedroom a sanctuary for sleep. Ensure your mattress and pillows are comfortable, and the room is dark, quiet, and at a cool temperature. Consider using blackout curtains, earplugs, or a white noise machine to eliminate disturbances.

Limit Exposure to Screens:

The blue light emitted by smartphones, tablets, and computers can disrupt your sleep-wake cycle. Avoid screens at least an hour before bedtime or use blue light filters on your devices.

Watch Your Diet and Caffeine Intake:

Avoid heavy meals, caffeine, and alcohol close to bedtime. These substances can interfere with your ability to fall asleep or stay asleep throughout the night.

Get Regular Exercise:

Engaging in physical activity during the day can improve sleep quality. However, try to finish vigorous workouts at least a few hours before bedtime, as exercising too close to bedtime can be stimulating.

Manage Stress:

High stress levels can lead to poor sleep. Practice stress-reduction techniques such as deep breathing, meditation, or progressive muscle relaxation to calm your mind before bedtime.

Limit Naps:

While short power naps can be refreshing, long or irregular daytime naps can disrupt your sleep pattern. If you need to nap, keep it brief (20-30 minutes) and earlier in the day.

Watch Your Liquid Intake:

Minimize the consumption of liquids in the evening to reduce nighttime awakenings due to bathroom trips.

Be Mindful of Light Exposure:

Exposure to natural light during the day helps regulate your circadian rhythm. Spend time outdoors in natural daylight, and in the evening, dim the lights to signal to your body that it's time to sleep.

Consult a Healthcare Professional:

If you've tried these strategies and still struggle with sleep, consider consulting a healthcare provider or sleep specialist. Underlying medical conditions or sleep disorders may require specific interventions or treatments.

Remember that improving sleep quality may take time, and consistency is key. By incorporating these strategies into your daily routine, you can gradually improve your sleep habits and enjoy the many physical and mental health benefits that come with a restful night's sleep.

SLEEP DISORDERS AND THEIR EFFECTS ON THE VAGUS NERVE

Numerous individuals suffer from sleep disorders that disrupt their normal sleep patterns. These disorders can have far-reaching effects on various bodily functions, including the vagus nerve, which is a critical component of the autonomic nervous system. This section aims to shed light on the relationship between sleep disorders and their impact on the vagus nerve.

The Vagus Nerve:

The vagus nerve, also known as the tenth cranial nerve, is one of the longest and most complex nerves in the human body. It originates in the brainstem and extends down through the neck, thorax, and abdomen. This nerve plays a crucial role in regulating various involuntary bodily functions, such as heart rate, digestion, and respiratory rate. It serves as a communication channel between the brain and various organs, helping to maintain balance and homeostasis.

Effects of Sleep Disorders on the Vagus Nerve:

Altered Heart Rate: Sleep disorders can lead to erratic heart rate patterns. Conditions like sleep apnea, where breathing intermittently stops during sleep, can cause an increase in sympathetic nervous system activity, leading to heightened stress responses and potentially compromising the vagus nerve's ability to maintain a stable heart rate. This can contribute to cardiovascular problems over time.

Digestive Issues: The vagus nerve plays a critical role in regulating digestive processes, including the production of stomach acid and the movement of food through the gastrointestinal tract. Sleep disorders, such as insomnia or disrupted sleep, can disrupt the vagus nerve's ability to coordinate these functions, potentially leading to digestive problems like acid reflux, irritable bowel syndrome (IBS), or even more severe conditions.

Inflammation and Immune Function: Adequate sleep is essential for maintaining a healthy immune system. When sleep disorders disrupt normal sleep patterns, chronic inflammation can result. The vagus nerve helps regulate inflammation by controlling the release of cytokines and other immune response mediators. Sleep disturbances can compromise this regulatory function, potentially leading to increased susceptibility to infections and chronic inflammatory conditions.

Mood and Mental Health: The vagus nerve also plays a role in mood regulation and mental health. Sleep disorders, particularly chronic conditions like insomnia or sleep deprivation, can contribute to mood disorders such as depression and anxiety. These conditions are associated with alterations in vagal tone, which affects the nerve's ability to regulate emotional responses and stress.

Autonomic Imbalance: The autonomic nervous system, including the vagus nerve, is responsible for maintaining the body's balance between the sympathetic (fight-or-flight) and parasympathetic (rest-and-digest) responses. Sleep disorders can disrupt this balance, leading to increased sympathetic dominance and decreased parasympathetic activity. This imbalance can have widespread effects on bodily functions and overall well-being.

In conclusion, sleep disorders can have a significant impact on the vagus nerve, disrupting its ability to regulate various physiological processes. This disruption can lead to a range of health problems, including cardiovascular issues, digestive disorders, immune system dysfunction, mood disorders, and autonomic imbalances. Recognizing the connection between sleep disorders and the vagus nerve underscores the importance of diagnosing and treating sleep disturbances to maintain

overall health and well-being.

CHAPTER EIGHT

LIFESTYLE MODIFICATIONS FOR VAGUS NERVE OPTIMIZATION

Holistic approaches to wellness emphasize the interconnectedness of the mind, body, and spirit in achieving overall health and well-being. Unlike conventional medicine, which often focuses solely on treating symptoms, holistic wellness seeks to address the root causes of health issues, considering the whole person and their unique needs. Here's a brief yet detailed exploration of holistic approaches to wellness:

Mind-Body Connection: Holistic wellness recognizes that mental and emotional well-being are integral to physical health. Practices like mindfulness meditation, yoga, and tai chi emphasize the importance of cultivating mental clarity, emotional balance, and stress reduction to promote overall health.

Nutrition: A fundamental aspect of holistic wellness is the emphasis on a balanced and nutrient-dense diet. Whole foods, rich in vitamins, minerals, and antioxidants, are considered essential for maintaining optimal health. Holistic practitioners often promote the consumption of organic, locally sourced, and minimally processed foods to support physical vitality.

Physical Activity: Regular exercise is key to holistic wellness. It not only helps maintain a healthy weight but also improves cardiovascular health, strengthens muscles and bones, and boosts mood through the release of endorphins. Holistic approaches encourage finding enjoyable physical activities, such as hiking, dancing, or swimming, to promote consistent engagement.

Holistic Therapies: Holistic wellness often integrates various alternative therapies like acupuncture, chiropractic care, and massage therapy. These therapies aim to restore balance and energy flow within the body and are used alongside conventional medicine to address a wide range of health issues.

Emotional Well-Being: Recognizing the impact of emotions on health, holistic approaches encourage emotional expression and the development of coping skills. Psychotherapy, art therapy, and support groups are tools for addressing emotional challenges and promoting healing.

Environmental Considerations: Holistic wellness extends to the environment, acknowledging the importance of clean air, water, and a toxin-free living space. Reducing exposure to environmental toxins and pollutants is seen as essential for overall health.

Spirituality and Connection: Many holistic approaches include a spiritual or philosophical dimension, recognizing the significance of inner peace and a sense of purpose in wellness. Practices like prayer, meditation, and journaling may be incorporated to foster a deeper connection with oneself and the universe.

Personalized Care: Holistic wellness is highly individualized, recognizing that each person has unique needs. Health practitioners in this field often take the time to understand an individual's lifestyle, genetics, and personal goals to create a tailored wellness plan.

Preventive Health: Prevention is a central tenet of holistic wellness. Rather than waiting for illness to manifest, holistic approaches emphasize regular check-ups, screenings, and lifestyle modifications to pro-actively maintain health.

Patient Empowerment: Holistic wellness empowers individuals to take an active role in their health. It encourages self-care practices like self-assessment, self-education, and self-advocacy, allowing individuals to make informed choices about their well-being.

Holistic approaches to wellness recognize that health encompasses more than just the absence of disease. They consider the entire person, encompassing physical, mental, emotional, and spiritual aspects of well-being. By addressing the root causes of health issues and promoting balance in all areas of life, holistic wellness offers a comprehensive and holistic path to achieving and maintaining optimal health and vitality.

CREATING A VAGUS NERVE-FRIENDLY LIFESTYLE

The vagus nerve, a vital component of the autonomic nervous system, plays a crucial role in regulating various bodily functions, including heart rate, digestion, and stress responses. Maintaining a vagus nerve-friendly lifestyle is essential for overall well-being. Here's a brief but detailed guide on how to achieve this:

Mindful Breathing:

Deep, diaphragmatic breathing activates the vagus nerve's calming response. Practice deep breathing exercises regularly, inhaling deeply through your nose, expanding your diaphragm, and exhaling slowly through your mouth. This practice helps reduce stress and anxiety.

Regular Exercise:

Engaging in regular physical activity stimulates the vagus nerve. Activities like yoga, tai chi, and aerobic exercises improve heart rate variability (HRV) and promote vagal tone, enhancing overall health.

Balanced Diet:

A diet rich in whole foods, especially fiber and omega-3 fatty acids, supports vagal function. Consuming probiotics, found in fermented foods like yogurt, also promotes a healthy gut-brain connection, benefiting the vagus nerve.

Hydration:

Staying properly hydrated is essential for maintaining optimal nerve function. Dehydration can lead to vagus nerve dysfunction, so ensure you drink enough water throughout the day.

Adequate Sleep:

Prioritize quality sleep to support vagus nerve health. Aim for 7-9 hours of restful sleep each night, as sleep disturbances can negatively affect autonomic nervous system function.

Stress Management:

Chronic stress can weaken the vagus nerve's responsiveness. Incorporate stress-reduction techniques such as meditation, mindfulness, progressive muscle relaxation, or spending time in nature into your daily routine.

Social Connections:

Meaningful social interactions and strong relationships have been shown to enhance vagal tone. Cultivate supportive relationships and engage in activities that promote social well-being.

Cold Exposure:

Exposing yourself to cold temperatures, such as cold showers or immersing yourself in cold water, can stimulate the vagus nerve and boost its activity.

Limiting Toxins:

Minimize exposure to toxins like excessive alcohol and tobacco, as they can negatively impact vagal function.

Intermittent Fasting:

Some studies suggest that intermittent fasting may support vagal nerve function by enhancing autophagy and reducing inflammation.

Positive Emotions:

Cultivate positive emotions through activities like laughter, gratitude exercises, and pursuing hobbies that bring you joy. Positive emotions can enhance vagal tone.

Biofeedback and Therapy:

In some cases, biofeedback therapy or other interventions under the guidance of a healthcare professional may be recommended to directly target and improve vagus nerve function.

Regular Check-ups:

Schedule regular health check-ups with your healthcare provider to monitor your overall health, as certain medical conditions can affect the vagus nerve.

Remember that creating a vagus nerve-friendly lifestyle is a holistic approach to well-being. Incorporating these practices into your daily life can contribute to improved physical and mental health, reduced stress, and enhanced overall quality of life. However, it's essential to consult with a healthcare professional before making significant lifestyle changes, especially if you have underlying medical conditions.

MINDFUL LIVING AND ITS BENEFITS FOR GUT HEALTH

Mindful living is a holistic approach to life that emphasizes being fully present in the moment, paying attention to one's thoughts and feelings, and fostering a deep awareness of one's physical and mental state. While it has gained popularity for its positive effects on mental well-being, it also holds significant benefits for gut health. We will explore the relationship between mindful living and gut health, highlighting how a mindful lifestyle can positively impact the digestive system.

Understanding Gut Health

Gut health refers to the balance and harmony of the gastrointestinal system, which includes the stomach, intestines, and the complex network of microorganisms that reside within the gut. A healthy gut plays a crucial role in overall well-being, as it influences digestion, nutrient absorption, immune function, and even mood regulation. An imbalance in gut health can lead to various digestive issues, autoimmune disorders, and mental health problems.

The Mindful Living Approach

Mindful living involves a range of practices that promote awareness, presence, and self-compassion. These practices include mindfulness meditation, mindful eating, stress reduction techniques, and regular physical activity. When applied consistently, they can positively impact gut health in several ways:

Stress Reduction

One of the key benefits of mindful living is its ability to reduce stress. Chronic stress can lead to inflammation in the gut and disrupt the balance of beneficial bacteria. Mindfulness meditation and relaxation techniques, such as deep breathing, can help lower stress levels, thereby promoting a healthier gut environment.

Mindful Eating

Mindful eating encourages individuals to savor each bite of food, pay attention to hunger and fullness cues, and make conscious food choices. This approach can improve digestion by allowing the body to better process nutrients and reduce the risk of overeating or consuming unhealthy foods that can harm gut health.

Improved Food Choices

Practicing mindfulness can lead to more thoughtful food choices. People who are mindful tend to opt for whole, nutrient-rich foods and avoid processed or high-sugar options that can negatively affect gut bacteria. A diet rich in fiber, prebiotics, and probiotics can promote the growth of beneficial gut microbes.

Enhanced Gut-Brain Connection

Mindful living fosters a stronger connection between the gut and the brain. This connection, known as the gut-brain axis, plays a crucial role in regulating mood and mental health. A balanced gut microbiome can positively impact brain function, reducing the risk of conditions like anxiety and depression.

Better Digestion

Mindful living encourages slower, more deliberate eating, which aids in better digestion. Chewing food thoroughly and being present during meals allows the body to produce sufficient digestive enzymes, making it easier to break down and absorb nutrients.

Mindful living is not just a philosophy; it's a lifestyle that can significantly benefit gut health. By reducing stress, promoting mindful eating, and encouraging healthier food choices, mindful living can foster a balanced gut microbiome and enhance overall well-being. Embracing a mindful approach to life can be a powerful step toward a healthier gut and a happier, more harmonious existence.

Dr. Chris Allan

CHAPTER NINE

CASE STUDIES AND SUCCESS STORIES

Over the years, several individuals have shared their inspiring real-life stories of how they improved their gut health by focusing on healing and optimizing their vagus nerve function.

Sophie's Journey to Healing: Sophie, a 32-year-old accountant, struggled with chronic digestive issues for years. She experienced bloating, gas, and irregular bowel movements. After numerous doctor visits, Sophie stumbled upon the connection between the vagus nerve and gut health. She started practicing deep breathing exercises and meditation to activate her vagus nerve's calming effect. Over time, her symptoms improved significantly, and she regained control over her gut health.

Mark's Battle with IBS: Mark had been battling with Irritable Bowel Syndrome (IBS) since his early twenties. The debilitating symptoms made his life miserable, limiting his social interactions and career prospects. Through extensive research, Mark learned about the gut-brain connection and its relation to the vagus nerve. He began incorporating stress-reduction techniques like yoga and mindfulness meditation into his daily routine. Gradually, his IBS symptoms subsided, allowing him to lead a normal, symptom-free life.

Emma's Remarkable Recovery: Emma, a 45-year-old mother of two, was diagnosed with Crohn's disease, a chronic inflammatory bowel disorder. Conventional treatments provided little relief, leaving her in constant pain and discomfort. Determined to find an alternative solution, Emma explored the potential of vagus nerve stimulation. She consulted with a specialized therapist who guided her through biofeedback and cranial sacral therapy, both of which helped regulate her vagus nerve. Emma's Crohn's disease symptoms improved, and she experienced fewer flare-ups, ultimately leading to a better quality of life.

John's Stress-Related Digestive Issues: John, a high-powered executive, suffered from stress-related digestive problems. His demanding job and busy lifestyle had taken a toll on his gut health. After researching the connection between stress and the vagus nerve, he decided to make lifestyle changes. John started practicing regular physical exercise, engaged in relaxation techniques, and prioritized sleep. As his stress levels decreased, so did his digestive issues, proving that a balanced vagus nerve can mitigate the adverse effects of chronic stress on gut health.

Lena's Battle with Anxiety and Gut Problems: Lena, a college student, struggled with severe anxiety and accompanying gut issues, including frequent stomach-aches and diarrhoea. Her therapist recommended a holistic approach that included psychotherapy, dietary changes, and exercises to stimulate her vagus nerve. Lena incorporated diaphragmatic breathing and progressive muscle relaxation into her daily routine. Gradually, her anxiety symptoms reduced, and her gut problems became less severe, highlighting the profound link between mental health and gut function.

Sarah's Journey to Gut Health

Sarah, a 38-year-old accountant, struggled with chronic digestive issues for years. She often experienced bloating, constipation, and abdominal pain, which affected her quality of life. After extensive research and consultation with healthcare professionals, Sarah learned about the connection between the vagus nerve and gut health.

Key Takeaways

Breathing Exercises: Sarah incorporated daily deep breathing exercises to stimulate her vagus nerve. Techniques like diaphragmatic breathing and the 4-7-8 method helped calm her nervous system.

Mindfulness and Meditation: Sarah practiced mindfulness meditation to reduce stress, which can impair vagal tone. This relaxation technique not only eased her anxiety but also improved her gut health.

Dietary Changes: Sarah adopted a gut-friendly diet rich in fiber, prebiotics, and probiotics. She learned that nourishing her gut microbiome positively influenced her vagus nerve function.

Within a few months, Sarah's gut issues significantly improved, and she experienced fewer digestive symptoms.

Khan's Battle with Gut Health

Khan, a 45-year-old IT manager, faced a lifelong struggle with irritable bowel syndrome (IBS). His symptoms included diarrhoea, cramps, and irregular bowel movements, affecting both his personal and professional life.

Key Takeaways

Regular Exercise: Khan began incorporating daily physical activity into his routine, which not only reduced stress but also enhanced vagus nerve function.

Cold Exposure: Inspired by the Wim Hof Method, John started cold showers and cold-water immersion. This unconventional approach increased his vagal tone and improved his gut symptoms.

Social Connections: Khan made an effort to strengthen his social bonds, as meaningful connections and positive interactions have been linked to vagus nerve health.

Over time, Khan's IBS symptoms became less severe, and he regained control over his gut health.

Emily's Holistic Healing

Emily, a 30-year-old yoga instructor, had a long history of gut issues, including acid reflux and frequent indigestion. Frustrated with conventional treatments, she explored holistic approaches to healing.

Key Takeaways

Yoga and Bodywork: Emily's yoga practice involved poses that targeted the vagus nerve, such as gentle neck stretches and backbends. She also received regular massages and acupuncture, which helped improve her vagal tone.

Gut-Brain Connection: Emily attended workshops on the gut-brain connection, gaining insights into how emotions and stress can impact gut health.

Nature and Grounding: Spending time in nature and practicing grounding techniques, like walking barefoot on the earth, improved Emily's overall well-being, including her gut health.

Emily's commitment to holistic healing eventually led to a remarkable improvement in her gut health, and she experienced fewer digestive discomforts.

Conclusion

These real-life stories highlight the transformative power of healing the vagus nerve to improve gut health. While each individual's journey was unique, the key takeaways underscore the importance of stress reduction, mindfulness, physical activity, and holistic approaches in promoting vagus nerve function and achieving better gut health. These inspiring stories offer hope and guidance for those seeking natural ways to enhance their well-being by nurturing the connection between their brain and gut.

CHAPTER TEN

PUTTING IT ALL TOGETHER - YOUR VAGUS NERVE-GUT HEALTH ACTION PLAN

Assessing the state of your vagus nerve and gut health can provide valuable insights into your overall health and help you make informed lifestyle choices. Here's a brief but detailed guide on how to evaluate and improve these crucial aspects of your well-being.

1. Recognizing the Importance of the Vagus Nerve:

The vagus nerve, also known as the "wandering nerve," extends from the brain-stem down to the abdomen, touching various organs along the way. It plays a central role in the parasympathetic nervous system, which promotes relaxation, rest, and digestion. A healthy vagus nerve contributes to better digestion, reduced inflammation, and improved mood.

2. Understanding Gut Health:

A healthy gut is essential for nutrient absorption, immune function, and overall well-being. The gut is home to a complex ecosystem of micro-organisms, known as the gut microbiota, that aid in digestion, produce essential vitamins, and help protect against pathogens. An imbalance in this microbiota can lead to various health issues, including digestive problems, immune disorders, and mood disorders.

3. Signs of Vagus Nerve and Gut Health Imbalance:

Digestive Issues: Frequent indigestion, bloating, constipation, or diarrhea can indicate both vagus nerve and gut health problems.

Chronic Stress: If you're under constant stress, your vagus nerve may be compromised, affecting your digestive processes.

Inflammation: Chronic inflammation in the body is often linked to poor gut health and can negatively impact vagal tone (vagus nerve function).

Mood Disorders: Anxiety and depression are associated with vagus nerve dysfunction and can be influenced by gut health.

Food Sensitivities: Developing sensitivities to certain foods can be a sign of gut health issues.

4. Assessing Vagus Nerve and Gut Health:

Heart Rate Variability (HRV): Monitoring your HRV can provide insights into vagal tone. A higher HRV indicates better vagus nerve function.

Gut Symptoms: Keep a journal of your digestive symptoms and note any patterns or triggers.

Stool Analysis: Consult a healthcare provider for stool tests to assess the diversity and balance of your gut microbiota.

Medical Consultation: Discuss your symptoms and concerns with a healthcare professional who can perform relevant tests and assessments.

5. Improving Vagus Nerve and Gut Health:

Diet: Consume a diet rich in fiber, prebiotics, and probiotics to support gut health. Omega-3 fatty acids, found in fatty fish, can also benefit the vagus nerve.

Stress Management: Practice relaxation techniques like deep breathing, meditation, and yoga to stimulate the vagus nerve and reduce stress.

Physical Activity: Regular exercise can improve vagal tone and promote gut health.

Sleep: Prioritize quality sleep as it plays a crucial role in overall health, including vagus nerve function.

Probiotic Supplements: Consider probiotic supplements under the guidance of a healthcare professional.

Social Connections: Engage in meaningful social interactions to boost vagal tone.

In conclusion, assessing and nurturing your vagus nerve and gut health is essential for overall well-being. By recognizing signs of imbalance, seeking professional guidance, and making lifestyle changes, you can take proactive steps to improve these critical aspects of your health and enhance your quality of life. Remember that the journey to better health is a holistic one, where the mind and body are interconnected, and small changes can yield significant benefits.

CREATING A PERSONALIZED HEALING PLAN

A personalized healing plan is a tailored approach to improving one's physical, emotional, and mental well-being. It is designed to address an individual's unique needs, taking into account their specific health goals, challenges, and preferences. Crafting an effective personalized healing plan involves several key steps to ensure its success.

Self-Assessment

Start by conducting a thorough self-assessment. Reflect on your current health status, including physical ailments, emotional struggles, and mental health concerns.

Consider your lifestyle, habits, and daily routines. Be honest and specific about your strengths and weaknesses.

Define Clear Goals

Identify what you want to achieve with your healing plan. Set specific, realistic, and measurable goals. Whether it's improving physical fitness, reducing stress, managing a chronic condition, or enhancing emotional well-being, having clear objectives will guide your plan.

Seek Professional Guidance

Consult healthcare professionals or experts in relevant fields. A doctor, therapist, nutritionist, or personal trainer can provide valuable insights and guidance based on their expertise. They can help you understand your unique health needs and recommend appropriate strategies.

Customize Your Plan

Tailor your healing plan to address your individual requirements. This may involve a combination of strategies, including dietary changes, exercise routines, therapy sessions, meditation, or medication. Ensure that these strategies align with your goals and are sustainable over time.

Establish a Routine

Consistency is key to success. Create a daily or weekly schedule that incorporates the elements of your healing plan. Make sure it fits into your lifestyle and is manageable. Gradually introduce changes to avoid overwhelm and maintain long-term commitment.

Monitor Progress

Regularly assess your progress towards your goals. Keep a journal to track your physical, emotional, and mental well-being. Note any improvements or setbacks. Use this information to make necessary adjustments to your plan.

Adapt and Evolve

Be open to adapting your healing plan as needed. Life circumstances, health conditions, and personal goals may change over time. Modify your plan to accommodate these changes and continue progressing toward your objectives.

Embrace Holistic Approaches

Consider holistic approaches that focus on overall well-being. This includes addressing the mind-body connection, such as practicing mindfulness, yoga, or tai chi. These practices can complement traditional medical interventions.

Engage in Self-Care

Prioritize self-care activities that nurture your physical, emotional, and mental health. Adequate sleep, a balanced diet, regular exercise, and stress management techniques are fundamental components of self-care.

Build a Support System

Share your healing plan with trusted friends or family members who can provide support and encouragement. Join support groups or seek out communities that align with your goals. Connection and accountability can enhance your journey.

Be Patient and Kind to Yourself

Healing is a process that takes time. Acknowledge that setbacks may occur, and it's okay to take breaks when needed. Practice self-compassion and celebrate your achievements, no matter how small they may seem.

In summary, creating a personalized healing plan is a dynamic and individualized process that requires self-awareness, professional guidance, and a commitment to self-care. By tailoring your plan to your unique needs, setting clear goals, and maintaining consistency, you can embark on a journey towards improved physical, emotional, and mental well-being. Remember that healing is a continuous endeavor, and adapting your plan as you progress is essential for long-term success.

………………………………………………………………………………

Special note to the reader:

Dr. Chris Allan
Wishes you good health!